Keto Clarity

14 Mistakes You Should Avoid While Following A Ketogenic Diet

Table of content

Introduction

What is a Ketogenic Diet?

The Ketogenic Diet, a diet traditionally used to treat pediatric epilepsy, has recently become popular as a means to lose weight. So what is a Ketogenic Diet, exactly? This diet is high in fat, low in carbohydrates, and moderate in protein. Most people see "high fat" and turn the other direction. Our society has been trained to believe that all fat is bad, and that all fat is inherently tied to weight gain, but this simply is not true of all fats. In essence, not all fats are created equal. This diet does not condone eating all trans and/or processed fats, but rather "good fats" such as omega-3 fatty acids and monounsaturated fats. Good fats can be found in foods such as avocado, nuts, olive oil, coconut oil, and eggs. You may have noticed that these foods are not overly processed, nor considered fast food.

How does eating more fat help you lose weight, when you are trying to also lose excess fat? The Ketogenic Diet is similar to a low carb diet in that one must avoid eating a lot of carbohydrates because carbs are converted into glucose. Thus, an excess of carbs effectively means an excess of sugar, which is then converted to fat stores in your body. The Ketogenic Diet forces a person's body to go into a state known as "ketosis" in which the body burns fats rather than carbohydrates. The ketones then replace glucose as an energy source, ensuring that there is no excess glucose floating around in your body to be turned into fat. Therefore, the recommended carb intake for those on a Ketogenic diet should not exceed 20-50 grams. This number can vary depending on your personal physical statistics and goals.

If you are not sure which foods are safe to eat for a Ketogenic diet, here's an example menu of a few days in the life of a person on a Keto diet:

<u>DAY ONE</u>

Breakfast:

Coffee with heavy cream, 1 tbsp of butter and/or 1 tablespoon of coconut oil

2 large, scrambled eggs with shredded cheese & 1 oz chopped onion

4 pan fried slices of bacon (yes, bacon!)

Lunch:

1 can of tuna

1 cup summer squash sauteed in butter or olive oil

1 cup of mixed greens with goat cheese

Dinner:

Buffalo Wings with sugar free blue cheese dressing

2 oz celery sticks

Snack Option:

½ avocado with salt and pepper

DAY TWO

Breakfast:

1 medium avocado with hot sauce, salt, and pepper

coffee with coconut milk and butter

2 slices of bacon

Lunch:

1 slice of chorizo quiche

I cup of cauliflower mash

Dinner:

Chili with pork, bacon, cheese, sour cream, diced tomatoes, tomatow paste, onion, green pepper, salt, pepper, and chilies.

Snack Options:

String cheese

almonds

<u>**DAY THREE**</u>

Breakfast:

"Fat Bomb" breakfast bar of pecan, almond, flax meal, and coconut oil.

coffee with coconut milk and butter

Lunch:

Chicken Enchilada Soup

Dinner:

Pork Tacos

Snack:

1 cup of chicken broth

Those starting the Keto diet may experience side effects such as fatigue, low blood sugar, dizziness, frequent urination, headache, sugar cravings, shakiness, muscle cramps, trouble sleeping, weakness, constipation or diarrhea, and/or heart palpitations. It is important to note that these side effects are *temporary* as your body enters a state of ketosis and becomes accustomed to it. After you achieve fat adaptation, you will no longer experience these unwanted physical side effects. This guide, however, offers 14 tips for avoiding mistakes that will lead you astray on the Ketogenic Diet. By recognizing these mistakes and correcting them, you are less likely to experience tiresome side effects, and more likely to achieve success in your weight loss and health goals. Remember to always speak to your primary care physician before starting any new diet.

Mistake 1 – Fat Phobia

Our society has trained us and ingrained in us the fear and avoidance of fat, no matter the source. Whether that fat be from fast food, processed treats, butter, eggs, olive oil, or nuts—we have been conditioned to believe that all fat is bad. But, as stately earlier, not all fat is created equal. The Ketogenic diet requires a person to eat low carb, which means that since you will be eliminating your main energy source, you *must* replace it with another energy source—fat. If you try to eat low carb *and* low fat, you will experience serious physical side effects that will not be healthy for your overall well being and health. Trust in your new energy source; and to do this, you must unlearn all that you have been drilled to dislike and know about fats.

So what fats *should* you eat? Fats such as saturated, monounsaturated, and Omega-3 fatty acids will set you on the correct path. At the same time, you should avoid vegetable oils and trans fats. Not sure how much fat to eat? Keep your fat intake around 50-60% of your daily calorie consumption; some sources even argue that a fat intake of 70% yields greater results. Through a few calculations and adjustments suited to your body's particular stats and needs, you will soon determine a number that works best for you. High fat foods that you will need to regularly eat to place you into this daily intake range include of lard, coconut oil, olive oil, and butter (a little bit in all of your meals).

Mistake 2 – Not Drinking Enough Water

On the Keto diet, people often first drop the excess pounds through the loss of water weight. Because this water weight will likely be shed through frequent urination, you will also inherently dispel your body's electrolytes. Make sure you are drinking enough water—even if you feel like you are bursting at the seams, to ensure that you do not experience unwanted side effects like headaches, nausea, etc. Other drinks such as chicken broth, coconut water, and low-sugar Gatorade (or another low-sugar energy drink) can also help to keep your bod hydrated during the ketosis process. The recommended daily intake for water is *at least* 50 oz, and even more if you exercise every day.

Mistake 3 – You Have A Cheat Day

Unlike other diets, a cheat day on the Ketogenic simply isn't possible. The Keto diet requires a set daily intake of fats to bring your body into a state of ketosis, which will take around 3-4 days (if done correctly). In the 3-4 day period of transition, your body will likely experience unpleasant side effects—physical ailments that you likely do not want to experience again so soon after achieving ketosis.

In a nutshell, if you have a cheat day you will bring your body out of ketosis. One cheat day effectively means a 3-4 day set back on your diet in which you will have to work to put your body back into ketosis. And with the unpleasant physical side effects, most will find that a cheat day just isn't worth the trouble. Do yourself a favor and don't get yourself kicked out of ketosis just so you can have that pizza on cheat day!

Mistake 4 – Too Much Sugar & Spice

You may be thinking you're eating low carb and high fat, but you're not seeing the results of ketosis in your body, nor the desire weight loss. The problem might be that you are actually consuming too much sugar. It is very important to look at the grams of sugar on every food that you eat so that you do not go over your daily intake amount and effectively negate all the work you have done.

Since carbs are converted to glucose, you must keep your daily carb intake anywhere from 20g to 50g. You should not be consuming any fructose from fruit or any added sugar from treats, soft drinks, processed foods, etc. If you are unsure if you have reached ketosis or not, it is advisable to purchase Ketostix. Ketostix are used to measure the level of excess ketones in your urine.

If you find yourself still needing a little sweetness in your diet, use Stevia, Xylitol, Sucrolose, Erthyritol, or Agave (use sparingly).

On the other side of the coin, too many spices can also be a hindrance in the Keto diet. What many people do not know is that spices have carbs! What's more, many pre-mixed spices contain unnecessarily added sugar. For example, it is advisable to use sea salt of table salt. Be sure to check the nutrition labels on your spices to get an accurate carb count reading for your daily intake. Spices high in carbs include cinnamon, bay leaves, cardamom, onion and garlic powder, and ginger.

Mistake 5 – You're Not Getting Enough Good Fat

As previously covered in this guide, on a Keto diet one should not be daily consuming fast food and processed foods high in trans fats. What's more, you may be eating the good fats, but are not incorporating them into *every* meal. You will first need to overcome the fat phobia, and then embrace the use of fats in every meal and snack (good fats such as saturated and Omega-3 and Omega-6 fatty acids). Good fat foods, that must be liberally consumed, include:

-**Avocados:** one avocado is about 77% fat. Avocados contain oleic acid, which is also found in olive oil. Avocados also have as much (if not more) potassium than a banana, and are high in fiber.

-**Coconuts and/or coconut oil:** Coconuts are made up of about 90% fat, making them a superfood for people on the Ketogenic diet. Since coconuts and coconut products are so high in fat, they help you stay fuller longer—therefore decreasing your appetite and increasing your body's fat burning mechanism.

-**Nuts, especially macadamias, walnuts, and almonds:** BE CAREFUL: peanuts, pistachios, and cashews are high in carbs so please consume these very minimally. Keto-safe nuts like almonds, walnuts, brazil nuts, and macadamias contain Omega-6 fatty acids and are high in fiber.

-**Chia Seeds:** A little-known underdog of fat-packing-power, just one ounce of chia seeds contains 9 grams of fat and are made up of about 80% of fat. Chia seeds are also high in Omega-3 fatty acids and fiber. Be sure to drink plenty of water when eating chia seeds, however, or you could become bloated and/or constipated.

-**Olive Oil:** Many people recognize olive oil as a superfood given its central part in healthy Mediterranean diets. Olive oil is loaded with antioxidants and vitamins K and E.

-**Full Fat Yogurt:** Don't be afraid of fat! Full fat yogurt contains probiotics, which help digestive health. You will certainly achieve your fat intake goals by eating this type of yogurt, but you must be extra vigilant about the added sugar. Many store-bought yogurts are, unfortunately, loaded down with excess and unnecessary sugars. It is advisable to stick with most Greek yogurts when on the Keto diet.

-**Eggs:** While some people may shy from eggs due to cholesterol levels, it is important to note that eggs are great for the Keto diet. 62% of one egg is from fat, and combined with the copious amount of vitamins and minerals, this food makes for a great fat to eat when on the Keto diet.

Mistake 6 – You're Not Taking a Supplement

Many people on the Keto diet will benefit from the consumption of one or more dietary supplements. These supplements can not only promote overall good health and well-being, but they can also cut down on the unpleasant physical side effects. While you do not have to take all of the following supplements, it is advisable to take one or two of the following—depending on your body's needs. Please discuss with your primary care physician which dietary supplements are best for you.

-Cod Fish Liver Oil: This supplement contains "good" fatty acids and will help with inflammation.

-Fiber supplement: Those new to the Keto diet may experience constipation and/or general digestive issues while the body adjusts to the new diet. This supplement will help regulate your digestive system and put it back on (working) track.

-Whey Protein (only for athletes): This supplement is only to be used by the extremely active, or athlete, person on the Keto diet.

-Probiotics: Those new to the Keto diet may experience constipation and/or general digestive issues while the body adjusts to the new diet. This supplement will help regulate your digestive system and put it back on (working) track.

-Potassium: If you feel like you're not eating enough avocados, bananas, or coconut, a potassium supplement may be beneficial on order to help with replacing your body's salt and electrolytes.

-Magnesium: Those new to the Keto diet may experience constipation and/or general digestive issues while the body adjusts to the new diet. This supplement will help regulate your digestive system and put it back on (working) track.

Mistake 7 – Eating Too Many Carbs

You may think you're eating correctly, but you may not be aware of hidden carbs. Remember to always look at the packaging of whatever you eat to get an accurate reading on your daily carbohydrate intake. Watch out for foods with hidden carbs such as spices, tomato sauces & products, peppers, and medicines like cough syrups. Obviously it should go without saying to avoid fruit, bread, pasta, chocolate (unless 70%-80% dark in small portions), milk substitutes, protein bars, salad dressings, baked beans, and barbecue sauce—just to name a few, in order to achieve success in the Keto diet.

Remember to keep your daily carb intake to around 20-50g per day, depending on your personal physical stats like height and weight—along with your goal weight.

Mistake 8 – Eating Too Much Protein

Recommended protein intake for the Ketogenic diet is around 0.8 to 1.2g/lb of lean body mass. If you are quite physically active, which you are likely to be if you are trying to lose weight, you will need more protein. This is why it is important to calculate your daily recommended protein intake from lean mass (calculated as total weight minus your body fat). You will need to know your body's fat percentage in order to calculate this ratio, which can be done using a tape measure or a caliper, or an online calculator such as: http://lowcarbdiets.about.com/library/blbodyfatcalculator.htm

As an easy rule of thumb, try to follow the 70/25/5 rule—that's **70% fat, 25% protein, and 5% carbs.**

Mistake 9 – Not Monitoring Sodium Levels

Low carb diets inherently mean low insulin levels, which in turn signals the body to shed excess salt and water. As mentioned earlier, the first level of weight loss on the Keto diet will come from water weight. In turn, you will be less bloated, but your electrolyte level will also be greatly depleted.

When you neglect the replenishment of your sodium levels, you will experience side effects such as headaches, fatigue, lightheadedness, etc. While we have also, to a degree, become as salt-phobic as we have become fat-phobic, you must remember to always add salt to each meal. Don't be afraid to put sea salt on your meals, or of making up a cup of broth with a bouillon cube and hot water as a snack.

Be careful to watch your sodium levels by paying attention to your body's physical reactions (or lack thereof). Keto dieters who do not monitor sodium levels may end up with a mild sodium deficiency.

Mistake 10 – Impatience

A lifestyle and diet change can take time, especially when you are essentially resetting the way your body processes food and energy. In the period while your body enters ketosis, you may become discouraged by the physical side effects. Following the steps previously laid out in this manual should eliminate some, if not all, of those side effects. It is also important to remember that our bodies will need time to adjust after a lifetime of consuming high sugar, processed junk foods. Giving your body time to adjust is key because fat adaptation on the Keto diet can take about one month. When fat adaptation happens, you are likely to experience a decrease in negative side effects and an increase in your energy and emotional well being—as well as weight loss.

Mistake 11 – You're Not Eating Enough Calories

When we think diet, we often think of the immediate restriction of food in general terms. And while this tactic may be true in some cases, the Ketogenic diet is not one of those times. As stated previously, dramatically cutting carbs means obtaining your energy from another source. In this case, you are getting the majority of your calories from fats. However, if you try to limit the amount of calories you are eating, you will inevitably become irritable, weak, fatigued, etc. What's more, limiting your daily caloric intake may actually end up hurting you.

Ever heard of the phase "eat little and often"? This saying applies to the Keto diet (and most other diets, really) in that eating too few calories can actually slow your metabolic rate. Metabolism is the chemical process in which the body breaks down foods in order to maintain biological functioning (living, essentially). When metabolism slows, the rate at which your body breaks down foods into nutrients—and thus breaks down calories, slows.

Like fat phobia, we must also break habits toward our manic calorie counting. Calorie counting is not only stressful, but it puts immediate walls and restrictions up at the time when you must nurture your body through the transition to ketosis, or to fat adaptation. By eating too few calories, you will essentially only hurt yourself and your weight loss plan.

This is not all to say that you should go into unbridled food consumption, as logical portion control is advised for most people. If you are unsure of how many calories you should consume, research the daily recommended intake for your weight, height, and gender. Most calorie counters also allow you to input your goal weight, so that you can determine how many calories you should eat per day in order to lose weight.

Mistake 12 – You're Focusing Too Much on Weight

Diets are often numbers driven, and so it is natural to want to get our scale out every day to track your progress. Here's a tip that will save you time, frustration, and impatience, as well as will break bad habits: put the scale away, give it away, or sell it!

Diets should *not* be about the number you see on the scale! Forget that myth. If you want to see tangible results, try to refocus your fixation on the numbers derived from waist, thigh, and arm measurements.

Not only is checking the scale unhealthy, but it also does not give us an accurate detailing of our weight loss. Have you ever weighed yourself in the morning and gotten one number, only to weigh yourself at night and gotten a number perhaps 5 or more lbs above the morning weight? This day-to-day, hour-by-hour fluctuation in our weights is natural, as it accounts for our meals, water weight, bloating, etc. That being said, the fact that our number on the scale is always in flux is very frustrating. Measurements are not only more tangible, but they are a more accurate determination of weight loss and health progress in general. For example, those with a lower inch measurement on their belly are often less at risk for heart disease or Type 2 diabetes.

Focusing too much on weight in any diet, or in any circumstance for that matter, breeds bad habits. Not only that, but it can also lead to more mistakes. By seeing a number that upsets you, you may take drastic action that can hinder your Ketogenic diet process. This is the point at which mistake #11 comes in with impatience. The Ketogenic diet process will ask us to unlearn many habits and lines of thinking, in addition to changing our eating routine. It is important that we are willing to learn, even willing to make mistakes so that we can progress in a positive and successful manner in order to achieve our goals.

Mistake 13 – You're Working Out Too Much

Too much of anything is never a good thing. While you should be exercising anywhere from three to four times per week, or at least doing some kind of heart rate-elevating activity for thirty minutes each day, you should also avoid over-exerting yourself.

When on a diet, we may have the determination to visit the gym everyday. For some people, that may be okay—their bodies may be able to handle that. But keep in mind that not everyone can handle training like an Olympic athlete—physically, mentally, or just plain having the time to devote to *that* much exercise!

Know your limits, while at the same time going out of your exercise comfort zone. Find what works for you in terms of time frame and how often you work out, as well as what type of exercise you do. It is very important, however, that on any workout regimen you must give your body time to recover. When we work out every single day and never give our muscles time to repair and revitalize themselves, our bodies simply will not be able to keep up. For example, if you tire your body out enough, you will not be able to carry on the seven days per week, multiple times per day work out regimen. Such a lifestyle simply isn't possible for anyone.

It's okay if you miss a day at the gym, or if you have to cut a work out short. Giving your body a rest is just as important as giving it a good work out. Striking a healthy balance is key.

Mistake 14 – You're Overeating

Where one person might restrict his calories, another might overload. It is important to note that on the Ketogenic diet, a person will feel "full" quite often. That's basically because fats are very filling. If by lunch you feel as if you can't possibly eat anymore, then listen to your body and either skip dinner or just have a light snack of nuts and/or string cheese. Essentially, don't feel like you *have* to overeat in order to achieve your macro limit (i.e. your daily fat gram intake). If you opt out of a meal on Keto and in turn, do not meet your fat gram limit—that's okay! We're all human. As long as you don't go *over* your daily intake of carbs, then your body will not get "kicked out" of ketosis.

As your body adjusts to the Ketogenic diet, you will begin to feel "less full" after each meal and snack. Remember, you are resetting your entire body's eating routine and in turn, you must give yourself time to adapt. This is where fat adaptation comes in. After you have achieved that state, it is less likely that you will feel full.

Sticking With It

When starting a Ketogenic diet, education is your greatest asset. Educate yourself on the science behind why and how the Ketogenic diet works. Educate yourself on which foods are okay to eat and which foods you must stay away from. Educate yourself on your body's specific needs based on your weight, height, measurements, and goal statistics.

For any diet or weight loss venture, ignorance is usually the cause of failure. If you do not know that X food has hidden carbs, but you are doing everything else right—how are you supposed to know what you're doing in wrong? This factor is why it is so important to check the nutritional information on absolutely everything that you eat. If you're not sure, or if the food does not include a nutritional information label, check the carb and fat levels of that food online.

One of the biggest hurdles with the Ketogenic is unlearning all your have been taught to abhor about fat consumption. What's more, you will need to train yourself to get the majority of your energy from fats instead of carbs. Following the 70%/25%/5% format, or a range close to this, will serve you well with staying on track and keeping your body in a state of ketosis.

As a bonus, here are 4 Keto-friendly recipes that can either start you out on the right track, or put you back on it:

<u>**Butter – Garlic – Cheddar Biscuits**</u>

Ingredients:

-6 ounces of cheddar cheese

-5 tablespoons of butter

-2 ½ cups of almond flour

-8 oz of cream cheese

-2 teaspoons of minced garlic

-2 teaspoons of baking soda

-2 large eggs

-3/4 teaspoon of xanthum gum

-1 teaspoon of sea salt

Directions:

First, pre-heat the oven to 325F and prepare a baking sheet. Next, mix 1 cup of almond flour and the cheese in a food processor. Combine until thoroughly mixed, then set aside for the next step. In a mixing bowl, combine the butter and cream cheese and microwave for 30 seconds—remove and whisk in eggs until the texture is smooth, then add the garlic, baking soda, salt, and xanthum gum. Next, combine the cheesy almond flour mix with the butter concoction, adding in the remaining measurement of almond flour until the mix becomes dough-like. On the prepared baking sheet, dollop on the dough about an inch apart. Bake the biscuits for about 25 minutes, or until the dough begins to lightly brown. Remove and let stand for about 10 minutes. Serve with butter and enjoy!

Cheddar-Bacon Quiche

Ingredients:

-6 large eggs

-1 cup of heavy cream

-4 slices of chopped bacon

-salt and pepper to taste

-8 ounces of shredded cheddar cheese

Directions:

Pre-heat the oven the 350F, then fry the bacon until crisp. While the bacon drains on a paper towel, whisk the 6 eggs together. Add in the salt, pepper, and heavy cream, then mix. Spray a 9 ½ inch glass pie dish, then arrange the bacon and cheese on the bottom. Next, carefully pour in the egg mixture over the layer of bacon and cheese. Bake the quiche for about 40 minutes, or until the egg begins to brown on top. Inserting a knife into the center and pulling it out clean will tell you if the quiche is finished baking or not. Let stand for about 5 minutes, then enjoy!

Goat Cheese Croquettes

Ingredients:

-1 lb of ground pork

-1lb of ground beef

-8 oz of goat cheese

-1 teaspoon of garlic powder

-1/2 teaspoon of cinnamon

-1/2 cup of chopped bacon

Directions:

Pre-heat the oven to 400F. In a large mixing bowl, combine together all the ingredients except the goat cheese. Next, create about eight 5 oz spheres. Make a pocket-type indentation in eat ball and then add the goat cheese inside each one. Seal the indentation with more beef-pork meat, then prepare a baking sheet. Evenly space out the croquettes on the baking sheet and bake for about 30 minutes. For a more crispy consistency, broil for another 5 minutes. Remove and let stand for 5 minutes before enjoying.

Keto-Friendly Peanut Butter Cookies

Ingredients:

-1 cup of vanilla whey powder (any brand)

-¾ cup of peanut butter

-2 large eggs

Directions:

Pre-heat the oven to 350F, then mix together the peanut butter, whey powder, and eggs. Stick the dough in the fridge for about 5 minutes if it appears too soft. Next, roll the dough into golf-ball sized spheres. Prepare a baking sheet with cooking spray, then place the cookie dough on it—evenly spaced. Bake the cookies for 5 minutes, then remove and let cool for another 5 minutes. This easy recipe will satisfy your sweet tooth in no time, without sabotaging your Keto diet!

Now that you have 4 great recipes to kick start your Keto diet, you are now well on your way to healthy weight loss. Since the Ketogenic does not have a calorie count like other diets, it is important not to limit yourself. If you limit yourself, especially being low carb, you will no doubt become weak, fatigued, dizzy, and/or nauseous. In turn, you must never try to be both low carb *and* low fat, as your body will never get the daily required energy it needs to operate at a healthy level.

Ketogenic diet calculators will be your friend in this process, such as http://keto-calculator.ankerl.com. By using a Keto diet calculator, you will be able to more accurately determine just what your body needs and doesn't need. Apps such as LifeSum and MyFitnessPal will also help with tracking your daily percentage of fats, proteins, and carbs.

Staying organized and educated will ensure your success on the Keto diet. And with this guide, you are now on your way to a mistake-free Ketogenic diet transformation. Congratulations!

Conclusion

Thanks again for downloading my book I would like to ask you a great favor in that you leave a short review of my book on Amazon if you enjoyed it—this would be most helpful. Take care and good luck on your journey towards a better lifestyle!

www.ingramcontent.com/pod-product-compliance
Lightning Source LLC
Chambersburg PA
CBHW070829260726
48654CB00024B/664